THE LOW FODMAP DIET FOR IBS

A Clear and Effective Guild to Understanding and Implementing Low Fodmap Diet and Finding Relief from IBS Symptoms

Grace Mitchell

Table of Content

INTRODUCTION

Welcome to a journey toward understanding and managing Irritable Bowel Syndrome (IBS) through the Low FODMAP Diet. If you are reading this, you might be seeking answers, relief, and a better quality of life. Whether you are newly diagnosed with IBS or have been managing symptoms for years, this guide is designed to provide clear, supportive, and practical advice.

Understanding Irritable Bowel Syndrome (IBS)

Irritable Bowel Syndrome is a common gastrointestinal disorder that affects the large intestine. The exact cause of IBS isn't fully understood, but it is known to involve a combination of abnormal gastrointestinal tract movements, increased sensitivity to pain in the gut, and disruptions in the communication between the brain and the digestive system.

Symptoms of IBS

The symptoms of IBS can vary widely in frequency and intensity but typically include:

- Abdominal pain or cramping that often decreases following a bowel movement
- Altered bowel habits (constipation, diarrhea, or a mix of both)
- Bloating and gas
- Urgency for bowel movements
- A feeling that the bowels are not fully emptied after going to the toilet

These symptoms can be intermittent and may be triggered by food, stress, or other environmental factors.

Impact on Quality of Life

Living with IBS can significantly affect your quality of life. The unpredictability of symptoms can lead to anxiety around travel, social events, and meals. Moreover, persistent discomfort and pain can cause frustration and emotional distress. Recognizing these challenges is the first step toward managing them effectively.

Introduction to Low FODMAP

The term FODMAP refers to Fermentable Oligosaccharides, Disaccharides, Monosaccharides, and Polyols. These are short-chain carbohydrates that are poorly absorbed in the small intestine and can be fermented by bacteria in the gut, leading to the production of gas. For many people with IBS, this fermentation process can exacerbate symptoms like bloating, gas, pain, and altered bowel habits.

How FODMAPs Affect the Gut

In susceptible individuals, FODMAPs draw water into the intestine, which can alter bowel movements and lead to diarrhea or constipation. Additionally, as these undigested sugars are fermented by intestinal bacteria, they produce gas, which can increase discomfort and bloating.

Goals of the Low FODMAP Diet

The Low FODMAP Diet aims to provide a clear path toward identifying which foods trigger your IBS symptoms. The primary goals are:

- ➢ To systematically eliminate high FODMAP foods that could be triggering symptoms
- ➢ To reintroduce them in a controlled manner to identify your tolerance levels
- ➢ To establish a long-term eating plan that is both enjoyable and keeps your symptoms at bay

This diet is not about deprivation but discovering a balanced way of eating that harmonizes with your body's unique needs. Together, through the chapters of this book, we will explore how to implement and personalize the Low FODMAP Diet, aiming for a life where IBS no longer defines your choices.

Embarking on this journey requires courage, commitment, and change, but you are not alone. We understand the complexities of dietary management and are here to guide and support you every step of the way. Let's begin this path to improved well-being together.

UNDERSTANDING FODMAPS

Definition and Types of FODMAPs

FODMAPs are a group of short-chain carbohydrates and sugar alcohols that are found in various foods, from fruits and vegetables to grains and sweeteners. The acronym FODMAP stands for:

- ➢ **Fermentable:** The process through which gut bacteria ferment undigested carbohydrates to produce gases.

- ➢ **Oligosaccharides:** Found in foods such as wheat, rye, onions, and garlic. These are chains of sugar molecules that are linked together in a way that makes them difficult to absorb fully by some individuals.

- ➢ **Disaccharides:** This category includes lactose, which is common in dairy products like milk and soft cheeses. Lactose can be particularly challenging to digest for individuals with lactase deficiency, a common condition that affects the ability to break down lactose.

- ➢ **Monosaccharides:** Fructose, a simple sugar found in higher concentrations in apples, honey, and high-fructose corn syrups, falls into this category. Fructose absorption issues can lead to symptoms when the amount of fructose exceeds that of glucose in foods.

- ➢ **Polyols:** These are sugar alcohols like xylitol, sorbitol, and mannitol, which are present in some fruits and vegetables and are also used as artificial sweeteners.

How FODMAPs Work in the Diet

FODMAPs are osmotically active, which means they pull water into the intestine, potentially leading to diarrhea in sensitive individuals. When these carbohydrates move into the colon undigested, they are fermented by bacteria residing there. This fermentation produces gases like hydrogen, methane, and carbon dioxide, which can cause bloating, cramps, and abdominal pain, particularly in people with sensitive guts or conditions like IBS.

Implications of FODMAP Intake

For individuals with IBS and similar gastrointestinal disorders, consuming high FODMAP foods can exacerbate symptoms. The key to managing these symptoms lies in understanding which types of FODMAPs trigger issues and adjusting the diet accordingly.

By reducing the intake of problematic FODMAPs, many individuals notice significant relief from their symptoms, enabling a better quality of life. It's important to approach changes in diet under the guidance of a healthcare professional to ensure nutritional balance is maintained.

The subsequent sections of this chapter will delve deeper into each type of FODMAP, exploring common sources in the diet and how they can be managed through careful dietary choices. This information is crucial for anyone looking to understand the impact of their eating habits on their digestive health and overall well-being.

Roles Of FODMAP in Digestive Distress

FODMAPs play significant roles in causing digestive distress, particularly for individuals with sensitive guts or conditions like Irritable Bowel Syndrome (IBS). Understanding these roles is essential for managing symptoms and improving gastrointestinal health. Here are the key ways in which FODMAPs contribute to digestive distress:

1. Osmotic Effect

FODMAPs are osmotically active substances, meaning they draw water into the intestine. This increase in fluid can lead to diarrhea in sensitive individuals. The extra water in the intestine can cause the bowel contents to move faster, leading to an urgent need for bowel movements and sometimes resulting in a loose stool. This aspect is particularly pronounced with high intake of monosaccharides (like fructose) and some polyols (such as mannitol and sorbitol).

2. Fermentation and Gas Production

When FODMAPs reach the large intestine undigested, they become substrates for fermentation by the gut bacteria. This fermentation process produces gases such as hydrogen, methane, and carbon dioxide. For people with a sensitive digestive system, this gas production can lead to an array of uncomfortable symptoms, including:

- Bloating: Gas accumulation can cause the abdomen to feel uncomfortably full and swollen.
- Abdominal Pain: The build-up of gas can create pressure within the abdomen, leading to cramps and aching sensations.

➢ Altered Bowel Movements: Excess gas can contribute to changes in bowel habits, such as increased frequency, altered stool form (loose stool or constipation), and urgency.

3. Changes in Gut Motility

The presence of undigested FODMAPs and the resultant gas production can affect the rhythm of gastrointestinal contractions, known as motility. Some individuals may experience an acceleration of gut motility (leading to diarrhea), while others may find their gut motility slowed (leading to constipation). The specific response can vary based on the individual's gut sensitivity and the types of FODMAPs consumed.

4. Visceral Sensitivity

Individuals with IBS often have heightened visceral sensitivity, which means they feel more pain or discomfort when their gut stretches from the gas produced during fermentation. FODMAPs, by increasing gas production, can exacerbate this sensitivity, leading to significant discomfort and pain.

5. Impact on the Microbiome

There is emerging research suggesting that FODMAPs can influence the composition of the gut microbiome. While FODMAPs can aggravate symptoms in the short term, long-term restrictions of FODMAPs might alter gut bacterial populations in ways that could impact gut health and immunity. This area of study is still evolving, and the long-term effects of a low-FODMAP diet on the microbiome are not fully understood.

Managing FODMAP Intake

For many people with IBS, a low-FODMAP diet can be a key strategy for managing symptoms effectively. This involves:

➢ Identifying and eliminating high-FODMAP foods from the diet temporarily.

➢ Reintroducing them gradually to determine personal tolerance levels.

➢ Establishing a personalized diet that balances symptom management with nutritional health.

It's recommended to undertake this process under the guidance of a healthcare professional, such as a gastroenterologist or a dietitian, to ensure that the diet remains balanced and that other potential causes of symptoms are adequately addressed.

THE LOW FODMAP DIET

Getting Started with the Low FODMAP Diet

Embarking on the Low FODMAP Diet is a proactive step towards understanding and managing your digestive symptoms. This diet isn't just about restricting certain foods; it's a journey of discovery, designed to identify what works for your body and to foster a harmonious relationship with your diet. Here's how you can confidently navigate the three critical phases of the Low FODMAP Diet: elimination, reintroduction, and personalization.

Phase 1: Elimination

The elimination phase is your starting point. This phase involves removing high FODMAP foods from your diet for a period, typically between 4 to 8 weeks. The purpose is straightforward: to give your gut a break and see if your symptoms improve without these potentially troublesome foods.

During this phase, it's essential to adhere strictly to the diet, as this is the only way to truly determine whether FODMAPs are the root cause of your symptoms. Foods like onions, garlic, apples, wheat-based products, dairy items with lactose, and certain legumes are excluded during this period.

Although it might seem daunting to restrict many common foods, this phase offers an opportunity for you to explore new ingredients and to discover the wide array of low FODMAP alternatives that are both nutritious and delicious.

Phase 2: Reintroduction

After the elimination phase, and assuming you've noticed an improvement in your symptoms, you'll begin the reintroduction phase. This stage is critical as it helps to pinpoint which types of FODMAPs your body can tolerate and in what quantities.

During reintroduction, you will methodically reintroduce high FODMAP foods, one group at a time, into your diet. For example, you might start by reintroducing foods containing lactose, like yogurt or milk, and monitor your symptoms for a few days. If you do not experience significant symptoms, you can conclude that lactose may not be a primary trigger for you and move on to reintroduce another FODMAP group, such as fructans found in garlic and onions.

This phase is highly individualized. Keeping a detailed food and symptom diary during this time is invaluable as it helps to track which foods trigger your symptoms and to what extent.

Phase 3: Personalization

The final phase of the Low FODMAP Diet is personalization. This phase is all about balance and creating a long-term eating plan that includes a variety of foods you enjoy while managing your symptoms. Based on the findings from the reintroduction phase, you can start to incorporate more high FODMAP food back into your diet, tailored to your personal tolerance levels.

This phase encourages flexibility and focuses on maintaining a broad, nutritionally balanced diet that doesn't restrict more foods than necessary. The ultimate goal here is to enjoy a rich, diverse diet that supports your overall health without triggering your IBS symptoms.

Throughout each of these phases, remember that the journey is uniquely yours. Each step you take is a learning opportunity about your body and how it responds to different foods. It can be empowering to discover that you have control over your symptoms through dietary choices. To ensure nutritional adequacy and receive tailored advice, working closely with a healthcare professional, such as a dietitian specialized in gastrointestinal health, is recommended.

By systematically working through these phases, you can develop a deeper understanding of your dietary triggers and lay the foundation for a healthier, more comfortable life.

The Importance of Working with a Healthcare Professional

When embarking on the Low FODMAP Diet, the guidance and support of a healthcare professional are invaluable. This specialized diet involves significant changes to your eating habits and can be complex, so professional guidance not only helps in tailoring the diet to your specific needs but also ensures you maintain overall nutritional balance.

Here are several key reasons why working with a healthcare professional is crucial when undertaking the Low FODMAP Diet:

1. Accurate Diagnosis and Assessment:

Before starting any diet for symptom management, it's crucial to have a correct diagnosis. Conditions such as IBS can mimic other serious health issues; therefore, a healthcare professional can help rule out other potential causes of your symptoms and confirm that the Low FODMAP Diet is a suitable approach for you.

2. Personalized Diet Planning:

Every individual is unique, and reactions to specific FODMAPs can vary greatly. A dietitian or nutritionist can help develop a personalized plan that considers your dietary preferences, nutritional needs, and lifestyle. They can also help you navigate the challenges of the diet, such as reading food labels, choosing suitable substitutes, and planning balanced meals.

3. Ensuring Nutritional Adequacy:

Eliminating a wide range of foods could lead to nutritional deficiencies if not managed properly. Healthcare professionals can ensure that your diet remains balanced and nutritionally adequate, providing alternatives and supplements as needed. For example, they can recommend appropriate sources of fiber, vitamins, and minerals that might be lacking due to the restrictions imposed by the Low FODMAP Diet.

4. Support and Motivation:

Changing dietary habits can be challenging. A healthcare professional provides not only expertise but also encouragement and emotional support throughout the diet. They can help you set realistic goals, celebrate your progress, and cope with setbacks. This support is crucial for maintaining motivation over the long term.

5. Monitoring Progress and Adjusting the Diet:

As you progress through the different phases of the Low FODMAP Diet, a healthcare professional can help monitor your symptoms and adjust your dietary plan as needed. This ongoing adjustment is crucial to identify the lowest effective dose of FODMAPs for your condition and to expand your diet as much as possible while still controlling symptoms.

6. Transitioning to Long-term Management:

Once your triggers are identified and your symptoms are under control, a healthcare professional can guide you through the transition to a less restrictive, more varied long-term eating plan. They ensure that this plan is sustainable and continues to meet all your dietary needs.

By involving a healthcare professional, such as a gastroenterologist or a dietitian specialized in gastrointestinal health, you ensure that your approach to managing your digestive health through diet is both safe and effective. This professional partnership empowers you to make informed decisions about your health and paves the way for successful management of your symptoms.

Foods to Avoid and Foods to Enjoy

Navigating the Low FODMAP Diet effectively requires a clear understanding of which foods to avoid and which to enjoy. Below, you'll find a comprehensive list that categorizes common high and low FODMAP foods. This guidance will help simplify your meal planning and grocery shopping as you manage your dietary needs.

High FODMAP Foods to Avoid

These foods are typically high in FODMAPs and may trigger symptoms in sensitive individuals. It's best to avoid these during the elimination phase and reintroduce them methodically to test tolerance.

Fruits:

- Apples
- Pears
- Mangoes
- Watermelon
- Cherries
- Peaches
- Plums

Vegetables:

- Onions
- Garlic
- Cauliflower
- Mushrooms
- Asparagus

- Artichokes

- Leeks

Legumes and Pulses:

- Chickpeas

- Lentils

- Kidney beans

- Baked beans

Dairy Products:

- Milk (cow, goat, sheep)

- Ice cream

- Soft cheeses (such as cottage cheese and ricotta)

Grains:

- Wheat and rye (in large quantities)

- Barley

Sweeteners:

- Honey

- High-fructose corn syrup

- Sorbitol

- Mannitol

- Xylitol

Beverages:

- Fruit juices (from high FODMAP fruits)
- Milk beverages
- Soft drinks with high-fructose corn syrup

Low FODMAP Foods to Enjoy

These foods are low in FODMAPs and are generally well tolerated. They can form the basis of your diet during the elimination phase and continue to be staples as you personalize your long-term eating plan.

Fruits:

- Bananas
- Blueberries
- Cantaloupe
- Grapes
- Kiwi
- Oranges
- Pineapple
- Strawberries

Vegetables:

- Carrots
- Cucumbers
- Lettuce
- Tomatoes
- Zucchini
- Bell peppers

- Eggplant

- Spinach

Proteins:
- Eggs

- Firm tofu

- Meats (such as beef, pork, chicken, and fish)

Dairy Alternatives:
- Lactose-free milk

- Lactose-free yogurts

- Hard cheeses (such as cheddar, Swiss, and parmesan)

Grains:
- Oats

- Quinoa

- Rice

- Gluten-free bread and pasta

Nuts and Seeds:
- Almonds (small servings)

- Macadamia nuts

- Peanuts

- Pumpkin seeds

Sweeteners:

- Maple syrup

- Glucose

- Stevia

Beverages:

- Lactose-free milk

- Herbal teas (without high FODMAP fruits)

- Water

Tips for Managing Your Diet

- **Read Labels Carefully:** Always check food labels for ingredients that might be high in FODMAPs. Manufacturers can change their recipes, so it's important to stay vigilant.

- **Portion Control:** Even low FODMAP foods can trigger symptoms if eaten in large quantities. Pay attention to serving sizes and listen to your body.

- **Diverse Diet:** Aim to include a variety of foods in your diet to ensure nutritional balance. Don't rely too heavily on any single food group.

By adhering to this list of high and low FODMAP foods, you can take significant strides in managing your symptoms and improving your quality of life. Remember, individual responses can vary, so what works for one person may not work for another. Keeping a detailed food diary during this process can help you and your healthcare provider understand your unique triggers and adjust your diet accordingly.

Strategies For Reading Food Labels

Reading food labels is an essential skill when managing a Low FODMAP diet, as it helps you avoid ingredients that can trigger IBS symptoms. Here are strategic tips for effectively navigating food labels:

1. Know the Common High FODMAP Ingredients

Begin by familiarizing yourself with the names of high FODMAP ingredients to look out for, such as:

- Fructose
- High-fructose corn syrup
- Honey
- Inulin
- Wheat, rye, barley (often found in processed foods)
- Milk, lactose
- Sorbitol, mannitol, xylitol, maltitol (sugar alcohols)
- Onion and garlic powders

2. Check the Ingredient List

Ingredients on food labels are listed in order of predominance by weight. This means that the first few ingredients make up the largest part of what you're eating. High FODMAP items appearing near the top of the list are likely to be in larger quantities, potentially causing greater issues.

3. Look for Low FODMAP Certification

Some products may have a Low FODMAP certification mark, indicating they have been tested and are considered safe for a Low FODMAP diet. These products can save you time and reduce uncertainty when shopping.

4. Beware of "Natural Flavors"

This term can sometimes include onion or garlic derivatives, which are high in FODMAPs. If a product contains natural flavors and doesn't specify what they are, consider contacting the manufacturer for clarification if you are sensitive to these ingredients.

5. Understand Serving Sizes

The impact of FODMAPs can be related to portion size. Check the serving size and compare it to the amount you typically consume. Smaller quantities of some high FODMAP ingredients may be tolerable.

6. Avoid Artificial Sweeteners in Processed Foods

Many processed foods contain artificial sweeteners that are high in FODMAPs, particularly the sugar alcohols sorbitol, mannitol, xylitol, and maltitol. Always scan the ingredient list for these sweeteners, particularly in diet foods and beverages.

7. Use Technology

There are several apps designed to help those following a Low FODMAP diet, such as the Monash University FODMAP Diet app. These can provide quick, handy references for identifying safe foods and ingredients while shopping.

8. Keep Updated

FODMAP research is ongoing, and recommendations can change as new information becomes available. Keeping yourself updated with the latest FODMAP research and lists will help you make informed choices.

9. Simplify Your Diet

Whenever possible, opt for whole and less processed foods. Fruits, vegetables, lean proteins, and grains that are naturally low in FODMAPs are easier to identify and don't require much label scrutiny.

10. Practice and Patience

Becoming proficient at reading food labels takes time and practice. As you become more familiar with high and low FODMAP ingredients, this process will become faster and more intuitive.

By applying these strategies, you can navigate grocery aisles more effectively, making informed decisions that support your dietary needs and help manage your IBS symptoms. Remember, individual tolerances vary, so what may be acceptable for others might still cause symptoms for you.

IMPLEMENTING THE LOW FODMAP DIET

Phase 1: Elimination

The elimination phase is the foundational step in your Low FODMAP journey, where you remove high FODMAP foods from your diet. This phase is crucial for resetting your system and identifying the foods that trigger your symptoms. Below are strategies for planning your meals, navigating dining out, and managing the challenges you may encounter.

Planning Your Low FODMAP Meals

1. Educate Yourself on Low FODMAP Foods: Start by familiarizing yourself with foods that are low in FODMAPs. Use resources like the Monash University FODMAP Diet app or consult with a dietitian to get accurate, up-to-date lists and portion sizes.

2. Create a Meal Plan: Planning is key to success. Design a weekly meal plan that incorporates a variety of low FODMAP foods to ensure nutritional balance and prevent monotony. Include meals that you can cook in bulk and use for lunches or dinners throughout the week.

3. Prepare Your Own Food: Home cooking gives you complete control over what you eat. Experiment with low FODMAP herbs and spices like ginger, mustard seeds, and chives to add flavor to your dishes without triggering symptoms.

4. Keep a Food Diary: Document everything you eat and note any symptoms you experience. This record will be invaluable for understanding your personal triggers and will be helpful when consulting with your healthcare provider.

Tips for Dining Out and Social Situations

1. Research Restaurants in Advance: Look up menus online before going out and identify places that offer Low FODMAP friendly options or dishes that can be easily modified.

2. Communicate Your Needs: Don't hesitate to explain your dietary restrictions to the staff. Most restaurants are willing to accommodate dietary needs if they are clearly communicated.

3. Choose Simple Dishes: Opt for dishes with straightforward ingredients that are easier to modify. Grilled meats and steamed vegetables are usually safe bets.

4. Bring Snacks: When attending social events, bring your own Low FODMAP snacks. This can help you avoid feeling left out if there aren't suitable food options available.

Dealing with Challenges and Setbacks

1. **Be Patient:** It's common to experience fluctuations in your symptoms during the elimination phase. Keep in mind that it can take time for your body to adjust to the new diet.

2. **Seek Support:** Join online forums, local support groups, or connect with others who are also following a Low FODMAP diet. Sharing experiences and tips can be incredibly helpful and reassuring.

3. Focus on What You Can Eat: Instead of dwelling on the foods you miss, try to celebrate the foods you can enjoy. There are many delicious Low FODMAP options that don't trigger symptoms.

4. Consult Regularly with Your Healthcare Provider: Regular check-ins with a healthcare professional can help you navigate the diet more effectively and adjust it as needed based on your progress.

5. Learn from Mistakes: If a certain food accidentally sneaks into your diet and triggers symptoms, use this as a learning opportunity. Analyze what went wrong and how you can avoid similar situations in the future.

The elimination phase is a time of learning and adjustment. By approaching this phase with preparation, patience, and a positive mindset, you can effectively manage your symptoms and gain valuable insights into the dietary choices that best support your health.

Phase 2: Reintroduction

After successfully completing the elimination phase, you'll enter the reintroduction phase. This phase is all about gradually reintroducing high FODMAP foods back into your diet to pinpoint specific triggers and determine your tolerance levels. This step is crucial for building a personalized diet that balances symptom management with dietary freedom.

Understanding the Reintroduction Process

The reintroduction phase involves methodically adding high FODMAP foods back into your diet, one group at a time. This process helps to identify which FODMAPs you can tolerate and in what quantities. Each food should be tested separately, typically over a three-day period, to observe how your body reacts without interference from other variables.

Keeping a Symptom Diary

1. Record Your Intake: Note down the specific food and portion size you reintroduced. It's important to maintain a low FODMAP baseline diet during this phase, introducing only one new item at a time.

2. Monitor Symptoms: For each food reintroduced, record any symptoms that occur. Symptoms to watch for include bloating, gas, constipation, diarrhea, or abdominal pain.

3. Rate Severity: Use a consistent scale (e.g., 0-5) to rate the severity of your symptoms. This will help you quantify your tolerance and compare different foods more objectively.

Reintroduction Schedule and Guidelines

Day 1: Introduce a small amount of a single high FODMAP food from one category (e.g., lactose, fructans). Observe and record any symptoms over the next 24 hours.

Day 2: If no significant symptoms occur, increase the portion size of the same food and continue to monitor and record any symptoms.

Day 3: If symptoms are still manageable or absent, consume a larger portion of the same food. This tests your upper tolerance limit for that specific FODMAP.

Day 4-6: Return to your strict low FODMAP baseline diet and monitor for any delayed reactions or lingering effects before introducing the next FODMAP group.

Tips for Successful Reintroduction:

- ➤ **Space Out Reintroductions:** Allow several symptom-free days between testing different FODMAP groups to ensure that any reactions can be clearly linked to specific foods.
- ➤ **Prioritize Foods:** Start with foods that you miss the most or that are important for your nutritional needs. This makes the diet easier to stick with long-term.
- ➤ **Be Methodical:** Resist the urge to rush this process. Accurate results depend on a careful and controlled reintroduction.

Adapting Based on Findings

Once you have tested various FODMAP groups, you'll have a clearer picture of which foods you can tolerate and in what amounts. This data allows you to:

> Gradually reintroduce more of the foods that did not cause symptoms.
> Limit or avoid those that did trigger symptoms.
> Customize your long-term diet to maximize both your gastrointestinal comfort and nutritional health.

Reintroducing FODMAPs can be a nuanced process, but it's a critical step towards understanding your unique dietary triggers and crafting a diet that supports your lifestyle and health without undue restriction. With careful monitoring and a methodical approach, you can gain the insights needed to manage your digestive health effectively.

Phase 3: Personalization

The personalization phase is the final and perhaps most liberating stage of your Low FODMAP journey. It's about using the knowledge gained during the reintroduction phase to create a flexible, sustainable eating plan that incorporates a broader range of foods while managing your IBS symptoms. This phase focuses on identifying your personal FODMAP thresholds and establishing a diet that you can maintain long-term, enhancing both your health and quality of life.

Identifying Your Personal FODMAP Thresholds

Your personal FODMAP thresholds are the specific amounts and types of FODMAPs you can tolerate without triggering symptoms. These thresholds can vary widely among individuals, which is why this phase is highly personalized.

1. Gradual Reintroduction Continues: Based on your observations in the reintroduction phase, you'll continue to experiment with incorporating FODMAP-containing foods into your diet. The aim is to determine the maximum amount of each FODMAP group you can tolerate.

2. Mix and Match: Experiment with combining FODMAPs to see how different mixtures affect your symptoms. It's possible that while you can tolerate certain FODMAPs well individually, your symptoms might flare when they are combined.

3. Adjust Based on Symptoms: Regularly assess and adjust your intake based on ongoing symptoms. Your tolerance may change over time, influenced by factors such as stress, hormonal changes, or other dietary shifts.

Creating a Sustainable Long-Term Diet Plan

1. Build a Balanced Diet: Incorporate a variety of foods from all food groups to ensure nutritional adequacy. Use the knowledge of your FODMAP thresholds to include as many high FODMAP foods as you can tolerate in moderation. This helps prevent nutritional deficiencies and diet fatigue.

2. Focus on Flexibility: Rather than a strict set of rules, your diet should be a flexible guideline that adjusts to your life's rhythms and changes. This adaptability is key to maintaining the diet long-term.

3. Keep a Symptom Diary: Even in this final phase, continue to track your diet and symptoms. This ongoing documentation can help you manage flare-ups and refine your diet further.

4. Plan for Flare-Ups: Develop strategies for times when your symptoms may worsen. Knowing how to temporarily revert to a stricter Low FODMAP regimen during flare-ups can help you regain control quickly.

5. Seek Professional Guidance: Regular check-ins with a dietitian can help ensure that your diet remains balanced and that you're not unnecessarily restricting foods. A professional can also help you adjust your diet plan as your lifestyle or health needs change.

6. Education Continues: Stay informed about new Low FODMAP research and resources. Ongoing education can help you make informed choices and feel empowered about your dietary decisions.

Embracing the Lifestyle

Ultimately, the personalization phase is about embracing the Low FODMAP diet as a lifestyle choice, not just a temporary intervention. It's about creating a relationship with food that respects your body's needs, enhances your health, and improves your quality of life. By now, you should feel more confident in your ability to manage your symptoms and enjoy a richer, more varied diet. Remember, the goal of the Low FODMAP diet isn't to restrict but to expand your choices by understanding your body better.

This personalized approach allows you to enjoy meals with fewer restrictions, participate more freely in social settings, and live without the constant worry of IBS symptoms disrupting your life. As you move forward, maintain a positive outlook, and remember that flexibility and mindfulness are your best tools for managing your dietary needs effectively.

BREAKFAST RECIPES

Low FODMAP Smoothie

Prep Time: 5 minutes

Total Time: 5 minutes

Serving Size: 1 smoothie

Ingredients:

- 1 cup lactose-free almond milk
- 1/2 ripe banana (unripe for lower FODMAP)
- 1/2 cup frozen strawberries
- 1/2 cup spinach leaves
- 1 tablespoon chia seeds
- 1 tablespoon maple syrup (optional)
- Ice cubes (optional)

Instructions:

1. In a blender, combine almond milk, banana, strawberries, spinach, and chia seeds.
2. If desired, add maple syrup for sweetness.
3. Blend until smooth.
4. If a colder consistency is desired, add ice cubes and blend again.
5. Pour into a glass and enjoy immediately.

Nutritional Information (per serving): Calories: 180

- Fat: 6g

- Carbohydrates: 30g

- Fiber: 8g

- Sugar: 16g

- Protein: 4g

Tips and Variations:

1. Substitute spinach with kale or Swiss chard for variety.

2. Add a scoop of low FODMAP protein powder for an extra protein boost.

3. Experiment with different low FODMAP fruits such as blueberries or pineapple.

Prep Time: 10 minutes

Cook Time: 20 minutes

Total Time: 30 minutes

Serving Size: 6 muffins

Ingredients:

6 large eggs

1/4 cup lactose-free milk

1/2 cup diced red bell pepper

1/2 cup chopped spinach

1/4 cup grated cheddar cheese (lactose-free)

Salt and pepper, to taste

Instructions:

1. Preheat oven to 350°F (175°C). Grease a muffin tin or line with muffin cups.
2. In a large bowl, whisk together eggs and lactose-free milk.
3. Stir in diced bell pepper, chopped spinach, and grated cheese.
4. Season with salt and pepper.
5. Evenly distribute the mixture into the muffin tin.
6. Bake for 20 minutes, or until the muffins are firm to the touch and cooked through.
7. Allow to cool slightly before removing from the tin. Serve warm.

Nutritional Information (per serving): Calories: 140

- Fat: 9g

- Saturated Fat: 4g

- Cholesterol: 190mg

- Sodium: 220mg

- Carbohydrates: 3g

- Fiber: 1g

- Sugar: 2g

- Protein: 12g

Tips and Variations:

1. Add low FODMAP herbs like chives or parsley for additional flavor.

2. For a meaty version, include cooked and crumbled bacon or ham.

3. Store leftovers in the refrigerator for up to 4 days, or freeze for longer storage.

Quinoa Breakfast Bowl with Pumpkin Seeds

Prep Time: 5 minutes

Cook Time: 15 minutes

Total Time: 20 minutes

Serving Size: 1 bowl

Ingredients:

- 1/2 cup quinoa, rinsed
- 1 cup water
- Pinch of salt
- 1/4 cup lactose-free yogurt
- 1 tablespoon pumpkin seeds
- 1 tablespoon maple syrup
- 1/4 teaspoon cinnamon
- 1/2 banana, sliced (unripe for lower FODMAP)

Instructions:

1. In a small saucepan, bring water and a pinch of salt to a boil. Add quinoa and reduce heat to low.
2. Cover and simmer for 15 minutes, or until all water is absorbed.
3. Remove from heat and let sit covered for 5 minutes. Fluff with a fork.
4. Transfer the cooked quinoa to a bowl.
5. Top with lactose-free yogurt, pumpkin seeds, maple syrup, cinnamon, and sliced banana.
6. Stir to combine and enjoy warm.

Nutritional Information (per serving): Calories: 350

- Fat: 9g

- Carbohydrates: 55g

- Fiber: 6g

- Sugar: 18g

- Protein: 12g

Tips and Variations:

1. Swap pumpkin seeds for walnuts or pecans if tolerated.

2. Add fresh blueberries or strawberries for extra flavor and vitamins.

3. Drizzle with a little more maple syrup if a sweeter breakfast is desired.

Prep Time: 10 minutes

Cook Time: 10 minutes

Total Time: 20 minutes

Serving Size: 2 servings

Ingredients:

- 4 slices low FODMAP sourdough bread
- 2 large eggs
- 1/2 cup lactose-free milk
- 1 teaspoon vanilla extract
- 1/2 teaspoon cinnamon
- 1 tablespoon butter for frying
- Maple syrup, for serving

Instructions:

1. In a shallow dish, whisk together eggs, lactose-free milk, vanilla extract, and cinnamon.
2. Heat a skillet over medium heat and melt the butter.
3. Dip each slice of sourdough bread into the egg mixture, ensuring both sides are well-coated.
4. Fry the soaked bread slices in the skillet for about 2-3 minutes on each side, or until golden brown and cooked through.
5. Serve warm with a drizzle of maple syrup.

Nutritional Information (per serving): Calories: 320

- Fat: 12g

- Saturated Fat: 5g

- Cholesterol: 210mg

- Sodium: 420mg

- Carbohydrates: 40g

- Fiber: 2g

- Sugar: 10g

- Protein: 12g

Tips and Variations:

1. Add a sprinkle of powdered sugar or a handful of low FODMAP fruits like blueberries or strawberries for extra sweetness and flavor.
2. For a dairy-free version, use almond milk and a dairy-free butter alternative.

Prep Time: 5 minutes

Cook Time: 15 minutes

Total Time: 20 minutes

Serving Size: 1 serving

Ingredients:

- 1/2 cup rolled oats
- 1 cup water
- 1/2 cup grated carrots
- 1/4 teaspoon ground ginger
- 1/4 teaspoon cinnamon
- 1 tablespoon maple syrup
- 1 tablespoon chopped walnuts (optional)

Instructions:

- In a small saucepan, bring water to a boil.
- Add the rolled oats and grated carrots, reducing the heat to a simmer.
- Cook for about 10-15 minutes, stirring occasionally, until the oats are soft and the porridge has thickened.
- Stir in ground ginger, cinnamon, and maple syrup.
- Serve warm, topped with chopped walnuts if using.

Nutritional Information (per serving): Calories: 270

- Fat: 4.5g

- Carbohydrates: 53g

- Fiber: 6g

- Sugar: 16g

- Protein: 6g

Tips and Variations:

1. Add a dollop of lactose-free yogurt for extra creaminess.

2. Increase the protein content by stirring in a spoonful of low FODMAP protein powder.

3. Substitute walnuts with pumpkin seeds for a nut-free option.

Lactose-Free Yogurt Parfait with Kiwi

Prep Time: 5 minutes

Total Time: 5 minutes

Serving Size: 1 parfait

Ingredients:

- 1 cup lactose-free yogurt
- 1 kiwi, peeled and sliced
- 2 tablespoons gluten-free granola
- 1 tablespoon maple syrup (optional)

Instructions:

- In a serving glass, layer half of the lactose-free yogurt.
- Add a layer of sliced kiwi, then a layer of gluten-free granola.
- Repeat the layers until all ingredients are used.
- Drizzle with maple syrup if desired.
- Serve immediately or chill until ready to serve.

Nutritional Information (per serving): Calories: 350

Fat: 8g

Carbohydrates: 55g

Fiber: 5g

Sugar: 35g

Protein: 15g

Tips and Variations:

1. Swap kiwi for any other low FODMAP fruit such as strawberries or blueberries.

2. For extra crunch, add chopped nuts like almonds or pecans, if tolerated.

3. Enhance flavor with a sprinkle of cinnamon or vanilla extract mixed into the yogurt.

Scrambled Tofu Wrap (Gluten-Free Tortilla)

Prep Time: 10 minutes

Cook Time: 10 minutes

Total Time: 20 minutes

Serving Size: 2 wraps

Ingredients:

- 200g firm tofu, crumbled
- 2 gluten-free tortillas
- 1/2 cup diced red bell pepper
- 1/2 cup spinach, chopped
- 2 tablespoons olive oil
- 1/4 teaspoon turmeric
- Salt and pepper, to taste

Instructions:

1. Heat olive oil in a frying pan over medium heat.
2. Add the crumbled tofu and turmeric, stirring to combine. Cook for 3-4 minutes until the tofu starts to turn golden.
3. Add the diced bell pepper and chopped spinach to the pan. Cook for an additional 5 minutes, or until the vegetables are tender.
4. Season with salt and pepper.
5. Warm the gluten-free tortillas according to package instructions.
6. Divide the scrambled tofu mixture evenly between the tortillas, fold, and serve immediately.

Nutritional Information (per serving): Calories: 320

- Fat: 18g

- Saturated Fat: 3g

- Sodium: 200mg

- Carbohydrates: 28g

- Fiber: 4g

- Sugar: 3g

- Protein: 12g

Tips and Variations:

1. Add a sprinkle of nutritional yeast for a cheesy flavor without the lactose.

2. For extra heat, include a dash of chili powder or diced low FODMAP chilies.

3. Serve with a side of lactose-free sour cream or a low FODMAP salsa for dipping.

Prep Time: 5 minutes

Total Time: 5 minutes

Serving Size: 1 serving

Ingredients:

- 2 rice cakes

- 2 tablespoons peanut butter

- 1/2 banana, sliced (unripe for lower FODMAP)

Instructions:

1. Spread 1 tablespoon of peanut butter on each rice cake.
2. Top each rice cake evenly with sliced banana.
3. Serve immediately and enjoy!

Nutritional Information (per serving): Calories: 280

- Fat: 14g

- Saturated Fat: 3g

- Sodium: 150mg

- Carbohydrates: 34g

- Fiber: 4g

- Sugar: 12g

- Protein: 8g

Tips and Variations:

1. Substitute peanut butter with almond butter if preferred.

2. Drizzle a little honey or maple syrup over the top for added sweetness.

3. Sprinkle with cinnamon or cocoa powder for an extra flavor boost.

Prep Time: 10 minutes

Cook Time: 5 minutes

Total Time: 15 minutes

Serving Size: 4 waffles

Ingredients:

- 1 1/2 cups gluten-free flour blend
- 1 tablespoon baking powder
- 1/2 teaspoon salt
- 1 teaspoon pumpkin pie spice
- 1 cup pumpkin puree
- 1 cup lactose-free milk
- 2 large eggs
- 2 tablespoons maple syrup
- 2 tablespoons vegetable oil

Instructions:

1. Preheat your waffle iron according to manufacturer's instructions.
2. In a large bowl, mix together the gluten-free flour, baking powder, salt, and pumpkin pie spice.
3. In another bowl, whisk together the pumpkin puree, lactose-free milk, eggs, maple syrup, and vegetable oil.
4. Add the wet ingredients to the dry ingredients and stir until well combined.

5. Pour the batter onto the hot waffle iron and cook until the waffles are golden and crispy.

6. Serve hot with additional maple syrup or your favorite low FODMAP toppings.

Nutritional Information (per serving): Calories: 310

- Fat: 12g
- Saturated Fat: 2g
- Sodium: 320mg
- Carbohydrates: 46g
- Fiber: 3g
- Sugar: 12g
- Protein: 8g

Tips and Variations:

1. Add chopped nuts or seeds to the batter for added texture.
2. Top with lactose-free yogurt and a sprinkle of pumpkin seeds for a nutritious twist.
3. Mix in a scoop of vanilla protein powder to increase the protein content.

Smoked Salmon and Spinach Omelette

Prep Time: 5 minutes

Cook Time: 10 minutes

Total Time: 15 minutes

Serving Size: 1 serving

Ingredients:

- 2 large eggs
- 50g smoked salmon, chopped
- 1/2 cup spinach, finely chopped
- 1 tablespoon lactose-free cream or milk
- 1 tablespoon chives, chopped
- 1 tablespoon olive oil
- Salt and pepper, to taste

Instructions:

1. In a bowl, whisk together the eggs, lactose-free cream, salt, and pepper.
2. Heat olive oil in a non-stick skillet over medium heat.
3. Pour the egg mixture into the skillet, tilting to ensure it evenly covers the base.
4. As the eggs begin to set, gently lift the edges with a spatula and tilt the pan to allow uncooked egg to flow underneath.
5. When the eggs are almost fully set, scatter the chopped spinach and smoked salmon over one half of the Omelette.
6. Sprinkle chives over the top and fold the Omelette in half.
7. Cook for another minute, then slide onto a plate and serve immediately.

Nutritional Information (per serving): Calories: 320

- Fat: 23g
- Saturated Fat: 5g
- Cholesterol: 370mg
- Sodium: 560mg
- Carbohydrates: 2g
- Fiber: 0.5g
- Sugar: 1g
- Protein: 25g

Tips and Variations:

1. Garnish with additional fresh herbs such as dill or parsley for enhanced flavor.
2. For a dairy-free option, omit the lactose-free cream or replace it with a dairy-free milk alternative.
3. Add diced tomatoes for a fresh, juicy flavor contrast (ensure they are deseeded to keep them low FODMAP).

Polenta with Roasted Tomatoes and Feta

Prep Time: 10 minutes

Cook Time: 30 minutes

Total Time: 40 minutes

Serving Size: 2 servings

Ingredients:

- 1/2 cup polenta (corn grits)
- 2 cups water
- 1 teaspoon salt
- 1 tablespoon olive oil
- 1/2 cup cherry tomatoes, halved
- 1/4 cup feta cheese, crumbled (lactose-free if available)
- Fresh basil leaves, for garnish

Instructions:

1. Preheat the oven to 400°F (200°C).
2. Place cherry tomatoes on a baking sheet, drizzle with olive oil, and sprinkle with a pinch of salt. Roast for 20 minutes, or until they are soft and bursting.
3. Meanwhile, bring water to a boil in a saucepan. Add salt and slowly whisk in the polenta.
4. Reduce the heat to low and cook, stirring frequently, until the polenta is thick and creamy, about 15-20 minutes.
5. Remove from heat and stir in a drizzle of olive oil for extra richness.
6. Spoon the polenta into bowls and top with roasted tomatoes and crumbled feta.

7. Garnish with fresh basil leaves before serving.

Nutritional Information (per serving): Calories: 250

- Fat: 10g
- Saturated Fat: 4g
- Sodium: 900mg
- Carbohydrates: 34g
- Fiber: 2g
- Sugar: 4g
- Protein: 6g

Tips and Variations:

1. For a protein boost, top with grilled chicken or fish.
2. Add sautéed spinach or kale for extra greens.
3. For a vegan version, substitute vegan cheese for feta and ensure all other ingredients are plant-based.

LUNCH AND DINNER IDEAS

Grilled Chicken Salad with Mixed Greens

Prep Time: 10 minutes

Cook Time: 10 minutes

Total Time: 20 minutes

Serving Size: 2 servings

Ingredients:

- 2 boneless, skinless chicken breasts
- 4 cups mixed greens (lettuce, spinach, arugula)
- 1/2 cucumber, sliced
- 10 cherry tomatoes, halved
- 2 tablespoons olive oil
- 2 tablespoons balsamic vinegar (ensure low FODMAP)
- Salt and pepper, to taste
- 1 tablespoon fresh chopped herbs (chives, parsley)

Instructions:

1. Preheat grill to medium-high heat.
2. Season chicken breasts with salt and pepper and brush with 1 tablespoon olive oil.
3. Grill chicken for 5 minutes on each side or until fully cooked and juices run clear.
4. Let chicken rest for 5 minutes, then slice thinly.
5. In a large bowl, toss mixed greens, cucumber, and cherry tomatoes.

6. Whisk together the remaining olive oil, balsamic vinegar, and herbs to make the dressing.

7. Arrange salad on plates, top with sliced chicken, and drizzle with dressing.

8. Serve immediately.

Nutritional Information (per serving): Calories: 300

- Fat: 15g

- Saturated Fat: 2g

- Sodium: 200mg

- Carbohydrates: 8g

- Fiber: 2g

- Sugar: 4g

- Protein: 35g

Tips and Variations:

1. Add a sprinkle of toasted pine nuts or walnuts for crunch.

2. Use lemon juice or a low FODMAP citrus dressing for a different flavor profile.

3. Incorporate other low FODMAP greens like baby kale or radicchio for variety.

Prep Time: 10 minutes

Cook Time: 15 minutes

Total Time: 25 minutes

Serving Size: 2 servings

Ingredients:

- 1 cup quinoa, rinsed
- 2 cups water
- 1 large carrot, peeled and diced
- 1/2 cucumber, diced
- 1/4 cup red bell pepper, diced
- 3 tablespoons olive oil
- 1 tablespoon apple cider vinegar
- 1 teaspoon Dijon mustard (ensure low FODMAP)
- Salt and pepper, to taste
- 2 tablespoons chopped fresh parsley

Instructions:

1. In a saucepan, bring water to a boil. Add quinoa, reduce heat to low, cover, and simmer for 15 minutes or until water is absorbed. Remove from heat and let sit covered for 5 minutes.
2. Fluff quinoa with a fork and allow to cool slightly.
3. In a large bowl, combine cooled quinoa, carrots, cucumber, and red bell pepper.

4. In a small bowl, whisk together olive oil, apple cider vinegar, mustard, salt, and pepper to create the vinaigrette.

5. Pour vinaigrette over the quinoa mixture and toss to combine.

6. Stir in fresh parsley and serve chilled or at room temperature.

Nutritional Information (per serving): Calories: 450

- Fat: 21g
- Saturated Fat: 3g
- Sodium: 200mg
- Carbohydrates: 55g
- Fiber: 8g
- Sugar: 5g
- Protein: 12g

Tips and Variations:

1. Add chickpeas or shredded chicken for extra protein.

2. Swap apple cider vinegar with lemon juice for a citrusy twist.

3. Include a handful of chopped nuts like almonds for added texture.

Low FODMAP Turkey Wrap

Prep Time: 10 minutes

Total Time: 10 minutes

Serving Size: 1 wrap

Ingredients:

- 1 gluten-free tortilla
- 3 ounces sliced turkey breast (ensure no high FODMAP seasonings)
- 1/4 cup shredded lettuce
- 1/4 cup sliced red bell pepper
- 1 tablespoon mayonnaise (ensure low FODMAP)
- 1 teaspoon mustard (ensure low FODMAP)

Instructions:

1. Lay the gluten-free tortilla flat on a clean surface.
2. Spread mayonnaise and mustard evenly over the tortilla.
3. Arrange turkey slices across the center of the tortilla.
4. Top with shredded lettuce and sliced red bell pepper.
5. Carefully roll the tortilla around the filling, folding in the sides to hold the contents.
6. Cut the wrap in half diagonally and serve immediately.

Nutritional Information (per serving): Calories: 320

- Fat: 15g

- Saturated Fat: 3g

- Sodium: 720mg

- Carbohydrates: 28g

- Fiber: 3g

- Sugar: 2g

- Protein: 20g

Tips and Variations:

1. Add a slice of lactose-free cheese for extra flavor and calcium.

2. Include fresh herbs like chives or parsley for added freshness.

3. For a bit of crunch, add cucumber slices or shredded carrots.

Prep Time: 15 minutes

Cook Time: 20 minutes (for rice)

Total Time: 35 minutes

Serving Size: 2 servings

Ingredients:

- 1 cup sushi rice
- 2 cups water
- 1/2 cup rice vinegar
- 1 tablespoon sugar
- 1/2 teaspoon salt
- 6 ounces sushi-grade tuna or salmon, diced
- 1/2 cucumber, thinly sliced
- 1 avocado, diced
- 2 tablespoons gluten-free soy sauce
- 1 teaspoon wasabi paste (optional)
- 1 tablespoon sesame seeds

Instructions:

1. Rinse the sushi rice under cold water until the water runs clear.
2. Combine rice and water in a rice cooker or pot, cook according to package instructions.
3. Once cooked, stir in rice vinegar, sugar, and salt. Let the rice cool to room temperature.

4. In bowls, evenly distribute the sushi rice.

5. Top with diced tuna or salmon, cucumber slices, and avocado.

6. Drizzle with gluten-free soy sauce and add a small dollop of wasabi if desired.

7. Sprinkle sesame seeds over the top and serve immediately.

Nutritional Information (per serving): Calories: 600

- Fat: 22g

- Saturated Fat: 3g

- Sodium: 1120mg

- Carbohydrates: 68g

- Fiber: 6g

- Sugar: 8g

- Protein: 32g

Tips and Variations:

1. Substitute fish with cooked shrimp or crab for different flavors.

2. Add thinly sliced radishes or shredded carrots for extra vegetables.

3. Include pickled ginger on the side for an authentic sushi experience.

Egg Salad Sandwich on Gluten-Free Bread

Prep Time: 10 minutes

Total Time: 10 minutes

Serving Size: 1 sandwich

Ingredients:

- 2 hard-boiled eggs, peeled and chopped
- 2 slices of gluten-free bread
- 2 tablespoons mayonnaise (ensure low FODMAP)
- 1 teaspoon Dijon mustard (ensure low FODMAP)
- Salt and pepper, to taste
- Lettuce leaves

Instructions:

1. In a small bowl, combine the chopped eggs, mayonnaise, mustard, salt, and pepper. Mix until well combined.
2. Toast the gluten-free bread slices to your preference.
3. Spread the egg salad evenly on one slice of bread.
4. Add lettuce leaves over the egg salad.
5. Top with the second slice of bread, cut the sandwich in half, and serve.

Nutritional Information (per serving): Calories: 400

- Fat: 28g

- Saturated Fat: 5g

- Sodium: 620mg

- Carbohydrates: 28g

- Fiber: 3g

- Sugar: 4g

- Protein: 12g

Tips and Variations:

1. Add sliced cucumbers or radishes for extra crunch and freshness.

2. For a spicier sandwich, mix a little low FODMAP hot sauce into the egg salad.

3. Swap out the lettuce for spinach or arugula for a nutrient boost.

Prep Time: 10 minutes

Cook Time: 0 minutes

Total Time: 10 minutes

Serving Size: 2 servings

Ingredients:

- 2 large red bell peppers, halved and seeded
- 1 can (5 ounces) tuna in water, drained
- 1/4 cup diced cucumber
- 2 tablespoons mayonnaise (ensure low FODMAP)
- 1 tablespoon chopped fresh dill
- Salt and pepper, to taste
- Lemon wedges for serving

Instructions:

1. In a mixing bowl, combine the drained tuna, diced cucumber, mayonnaise, and fresh dill. Season with salt and pepper to taste.
2. Mix thoroughly until all ingredients are well combined.
3. Spoon the tuna mixture evenly into the halved bell peppers.
4. Serve immediately with a lemon wedge to squeeze over the top.

Nutritional Information (per serving): Calories: 180

- Fat: 8g

- Saturated Fat: 1.5g

- Sodium: 290mg

- Carbohydrates: 10g

- Fiber: 3g

- Sugar: 6g

- Protein: 20g

Tips and Variations:

1. For a spicy kick, add a few drops of low FODMAP hot sauce to the tuna mixture.

2. Substitute tuna with canned chicken or salmon for a different protein option.

3. Add chopped olives or capers for extra flavor, ensuring they are low FODMAP safe.

Rice Noodle Bowl with Ginger Lime Dressing

Prep Time: 15 minutes

Cook Time: 5 minutes

Total Time: 20 minutes

Serving Size: 2 servings

Ingredients:

- 200g rice noodles
- 1 carrot, julienned
- 1/2 cucumber, julienned
- 1/4 cup chopped green onions (green parts only)
- 1/4 cup chopped fresh cilantro
- For the Dressing:
- 2 tablespoons lime juice
- 1 tablespoon grated ginger
- 2 tablespoons soy sauce (gluten-free)
- 1 teaspoon sugar
- 2 tablespoons sesame oil

Instructions:

1. Cook rice noodles according to package instructions, then rinse under cold water and drain.

2. In a large bowl, combine the cooked noodles, julienned carrot, cucumber, green onions, and cilantro.

3. In a small bowl, whisk together lime juice, grated ginger, soy sauce, sugar, and sesame oil to make the dressing.

4. Pour the dressing over the noodle mixture and toss well to coat.

5. Serve the noodle bowl chilled or at room temperature.

Nutritional Information (per serving): Calories: 420

- Fat: 14g
- Saturated Fat: 2g
- Sodium: 640mg
- Carbohydrates: 66g
- Fiber: 3g
- Sugar: 5g
- Protein: 8g

Tips and Variations:

1. Add cooked shrimp or chicken for a protein boost.

2. Top with chopped peanuts or sesame seeds for added crunch (ensure tolerance for nuts).

3. Include bell pepper strips for additional color and crunch.

Zucchini Noodle Salad with Grilled Shrimp

Prep Time: 15 minutes

Cook Time: 10 minutes

Total Time: 25 minutes

Serving Size: 2 servings

Ingredients:

-   2 medium zucchinis, spiralized
-   12 large shrimp, peeled and deveined
-   1 tablespoon olive oil
-   Salt and pepper, to taste

For the Dressing:

-   2 tablespoons lemon juice
-   1 garlic clove, minced (optional, depending on tolerance)
-   1 teaspoon Dijon mustard (ensure low FODMAP)
-   3 tablespoons olive oil
-   Salt and pepper, to taste

Instructions:

1. Preheat the grill to medium-high heat.
2. Toss the shrimp with 1 tablespoon olive oil, salt, and pepper.
3. Grill the shrimp for 2-3 minutes per side or until they are pink and opaque.
4. In a large bowl, combine the spiralized zucchini.
5. For the dressing, whisk together lemon juice, minced garlic (if using), Dijon mustard, and 3 tablespoons olive oil in a small bowl. Season with salt and pepper.

6. Pour the dressing over the zucchini noodles and toss to coat.

7. Top the zucchini noodles with grilled shrimp and serve immediately.

Nutritional Information (per serving): Calories: 320

- Fat: 22g

- Saturated Fat: 3g

- Sodium: 300mg

- Carbohydrates: 10g

- Fiber: 2g

- Sugar: 6g

- Protein: 20g

Tips and Variations:

1. For a non-seafood version, substitute grilled chicken or tofu.

2. Add cherry tomatoes or sliced radishes for extra color and texture.

3. Sprinkle with chopped fresh basil or parsley for a fresh herb finish.

Prep Time: 15 minutes

Cook Time: 40 minutes

Total Time: 55 minutes

Serving Size: 2 servings

Ingredients:

- 2 medium eggplants
- 1 cup cooked rice
- 1/4 cup diced red bell pepper
- 1/4 cup chopped fresh parsley
- 1/4 cup chopped fresh basil
- 2 tablespoons olive oil
- Salt and pepper, to taste
- 1/4 cup crumbled feta cheese (lactose-free if available)

Instructions:

1. Preheat the oven to 375°F (190°C).
2. Cut the eggplants in half lengthwise. Scoop out the centers, leaving a thin shell, and chop the removed eggplant flesh.
3. In a skillet, heat 1 tablespoon of olive oil over medium heat. Sauté the chopped eggplant flesh and red bell pepper until softened, about 5-7 minutes.
4. Remove from heat and mix in the cooked rice, parsley, basil, and half of the feta cheese. Season with salt and pepper.
5. Stuff the eggplant halves with the rice mixture and place them in a baking dish.

6. Drizzle with the remaining olive oil and sprinkle the rest of the feta cheese over the top.

7. Cover with foil and bake for 30 minutes. Remove the foil and bake for an additional 10 minutes, or until the eggplants are tender and the topping is golden.

8. Serve warm.

Nutritional Information (per serving): Calories: 320

- Fat: 18g
- Saturated Fat: 5g
- Sodium: 300mg
- Carbohydrates: 36g
- Fiber: 9g
- Sugar: 13g
- Protein: 8g

Tips and Variations:

1. Add pine nuts or chopped walnuts for a crunchy texture.
2. For added protein, mix in some cooked ground turkey or quinoa with the rice filling.
3. Substitute feta with grated Parmesan for a different flavor profile.

Prep Time: 10 minutes

Total Time: 10 minutes

Serving Size: 2 servings

Ingredients:

- 3 cups chopped romaine lettuce
- 1/2 cucumber, sliced
- 10 cherry tomatoes, halved
- 1/4 cup sliced black olives (ensure low FODMAP and drained)
- 1/4 red bell pepper, sliced
- 1/4 cup crumbled lactose-free feta cheese
- 2 tablespoons olive oil
- 1 tablespoon red wine vinegar
- Salt and pepper, to taste

Instructions:

1. In a large salad bowl, combine romaine lettuce, cucumber, cherry tomatoes, black olives, and red bell pepper.
2. Sprinkle crumbled feta cheese over the top.
3. In a small bowl, whisk together olive oil and red wine vinegar. Season with salt and pepper.
4. Drizzle the dressing over the salad and toss gently to combine.
5. Serve immediately.

Nutritional Information (per serving): Calories: 250

- Fat: 21g

- Saturated Fat: 5g

- Sodium: 380mg

- Carbohydrates: 12g

- Fiber: 3g

- Sugar: 5g

- Protein: 5g

Tips and Variations:

1. Add a protein such as grilled chicken or tofu to make it a heartier meal.

2. Include a sprinkle of dried oregano for an authentic Greek flavor.

3. Serve with a side of low FODMAP garlic-infused olive oil for extra dipping.

Lemon Herb Tilapia with Steamed Green Beans

Prep Time: 5 minutes

Cook Time: 15 minutes

Total Time: 20 minutes

Serving Size: 2 servings

Ingredients:

- 2 tilapia fillets (about 6 ounces each)
- Juice of 1 lemon
- 2 tablespoons olive oil
- 1 tablespoon chopped fresh parsley
- 1 tablespoon chopped fresh dill
- Salt and pepper, to taste
- 1 cup green beans, trimmed

Instructions:

1. Preheat the oven to 400°F (200°C).
2. Place tilapia fillets in a baking dish. Drizzle with olive oil and lemon juice.
3. Sprinkle chopped parsley, dill, salt, and pepper over the fillets.
4. Arrange green beans around the fish in the baking dish.
5. Bake in the preheated oven for 12-15 minutes, or until the fish flakes easily with a fork and the green beans are tender.
6. Serve the tilapia and green beans hot, garnished with lemon slices.

Nutritional Information (per serving): Calories: 280

- Fat: 15g

- Saturated Fat: 2g

- Sodium: 120mg

- Carbohydrates: 6g

- Fiber: 2g

- Sugar: 1g

- Protein: 31g

Tips and Variations:

1. Substitute tilapia with other mild white fish like cod or haddock.

2. Mix in some capers or sliced olives with the green beans for added zest.

3. For extra lemon flavor, include lemon zest in the herb mixture before baking.

Prep Time: 10 minutes

Cook Time: 20 minutes

Total Time: 30 minutes

Serving Size: 2 servings

Ingredients:

- 2 salmon fillets (6 ounces each)
- 1/4 cup maple syrup
- 1 tablespoon Dijon mustard (ensure low FODMAP)
- 1 tablespoon olive oil
- Salt and pepper, to taste
- 1 cup quinoa
- 2 cups water
- 1 cup carrots, sliced

Instructions:

1. Preheat the oven to 375°F (190°C).
2. In a small bowl, whisk together maple syrup, Dijon mustard, and a pinch of salt and pepper.
3. Place salmon fillets on a baking sheet lined with parchment paper. Brush each fillet with the maple syrup mixture.
4. Bake in the preheated oven for 15-20 minutes, or until salmon is cooked through and flakes easily with a fork.

5. While the salmon is baking, rinse quinoa under cold water. Add quinoa and water to a saucepan and bring to a boil. Reduce heat to low, cover, and simmer for 15 minutes, or until water is absorbed.

6. In another pan, heat olive oil over medium heat. Add sliced carrots and sauté until tender, about 8-10 minutes.

7. Serve salmon over a bed of quinoa and side of sautéed carrots.

Nutritional Information (per serving): Calories: 600

- Fat: 22g
- Saturated Fat: 3g
- Sodium: 200mg
- Carbohydrates: 58g
- Fiber: 5g
- Sugar: 15g
- Protein: 35g

Tips and Variations:

1. Garnish with fresh parsley or dill for an extra touch of flavor.
2. Swap quinoa for brown rice if preferred or for variety.
3. Add a squeeze of fresh lemon juice to the salmon before serving for added zing.

Vegetarian Chili with Canned Chickpeas

Prep Time: 10 minutes

Cook Time: 30 minutes

Total Time: 40 minutes

Serving Size: 4 servings

Ingredients:

- 1 can (15 ounces) chickpeas, rinsed and drained
- 1 can (15 ounces) diced tomatoes (no added high FODMAP ingredients)
- 1 cup water
- 1 carrot, diced
- 1 bell pepper, diced
- 1 zucchini, diced
- 1 teaspoon cumin
- 1 teaspoon smoked paprika
- Salt and pepper, to taste
- 2 tablespoons olive oil
- Fresh cilantro, chopped for garnish

Instructions:

1. Heat olive oil in a large pot over medium heat.
2. Add diced carrot, bell pepper, and zucchini, sautéing until vegetables begin to soften, about 5-7 minutes.
3. Stir in cumin, smoked paprika, salt, and pepper.
4. Add canned tomatoes, chickpeas, and water. Bring the mixture to a simmer.

5. Reduce heat and let simmer for 20-25 minutes, stirring occasionally.

6. Serve hot, garnished with fresh cilantro.

Nutritional Information (per serving): Calories: 250

- Fat: 8g

- Saturated Fat: 1g

- Sodium: 300mg

- Carbohydrates: 36g

- Fiber: 9g

- Sugar: 8g

- Protein: 10g

Tips and Variations:

1. For a spicy kick, add a pinch of chili powder or a dash of hot sauce.

2. Include a dollop of lactose-free sour cream or Greek yogurt on top before serving.

3. If tolerated, add a small amount of diced celery for additional flavor and crunch.

Prep Time: 10 minutes

Cook Time: 20 minutes

Total Time: 30 minutes

Serving Size: 2 servings

Ingredients:

- 12 large sea scallops
- 1 cup polenta (corn grits)
- 4 cups water
- 1 tablespoon olive oil
- 2 cups spinach leaves
- Salt and pepper, to taste
- Lemon wedges, for serving

Instructions:

1. Rinse scallops and pat dry with paper towels. Season with salt and pepper.
2. Heat olive oil in a large skillet over high heat. Add scallops, searing until golden brown on each side and cooked through, about 2-3 minutes per side.
3. In a saucepan, bring water to a boil. Gradually whisk in polenta and reduce heat to low. Cook, stirring frequently, until polenta is creamy and thickened, about 15-20 minutes.
4. In the last few minutes of cooking the polenta, stir in the spinach until wilted.
5. Serve scallops over a bed of creamy polenta and spinach. Squeeze fresh lemon over the dish before serving.

Nutritional Information (per serving): Calories: 450

- Fat: 9g

- Saturated Fat: 1.5g

- Sodium: 550mg

- Carbohydrates: 65g

- Fiber: 4g

- Sugar: 2g

- Protein: 30g

Tips and Variations:

1. Garnish with chopped parsley or chives for a burst of color and flavor.

2. For an extra creamy polenta, stir in a tablespoon of butter or lactose-free cream cheese at the end of cooking.

3. Replace spinach with kale or another leafy green if desired.

Prep Time: 10 minutes

Cook Time: 15 minutes

Total Time: 25 minutes

Serving Size: 2 servings

Ingredients:

- 2 cod fillets (6 ounces each)
- 1/2 cup gluten-free breadcrumbs
- 2 tablespoons grated Parmesan cheese (ensure lactose-free if sensitive)
- 1 tablespoon fresh chopped parsley
- 1 teaspoon lemon zest
- 1 clove garlic, minced (optional, omit if sensitive)
- 2 tablespoons olive oil
- Salt and pepper, to taste
- Lemon wedges, for serving

Instructions:

1. Preheat the oven to 400°F (200°C). Line a baking sheet with parchment paper.
2. In a small bowl, mix together gluten-free breadcrumbs, Parmesan cheese, chopped parsley, lemon zest, and minced garlic (if using). Drizzle with 1 tablespoon olive oil and mix until the mixture is crumbly.
3. Place cod fillets on the prepared baking sheet. Brush each fillet with the remaining olive oil and season with salt and pepper.

4. Press the breadcrumb mixture onto the top of each cod fillet, covering them evenly.

5. Bake in the preheated oven for 12-15 minutes, or until the crust is golden and the fish flakes easily with a fork.

6. Serve immediately with lemon wedges on the side.

Nutritional Information (per serving): Calories: 310

- Fat: 15g
- Saturated Fat: 3g
- Sodium: 200mg
- Carbohydrates: 10g
- Fiber: 1g
- Sugar: 1g
- Protein: 35g

Tips and Variations:

1. Substitute cod with another firm white fish like haddock or tilapia.

2. Add crushed almonds or walnuts to the breadcrumb mix for extra crunch.

3. For a citrus twist, replace lemon zest with orange zest.

Prep Time: 15 minutes

Cook Time: 45 minutes

Total Time: 1 hour

Serving Size: 4 servings

Ingredients:

- 1 tablespoon olive oil
- 2 chicken breasts, cut into chunks (can substitute with firm tofu for a vegetarian option)
- 1 bell pepper, chopped
- 1 carrot, peeled and sliced
- 1 zucchini, chopped
- 2 cups canned diced tomatoes (ensure no onion or garlic)
- 1 teaspoon ground cumin
- 1 teaspoon ground coriander
- 1 teaspoon paprika
- 1/2 teaspoon ground cinnamon
- 2 cups water
- 1 cup quinoa
- Salt and pepper, to taste
- Fresh cilantro, chopped for garnish

Instructions:

1. Heat olive oil in a large pot over medium heat. Add chicken chunks and brown them, about 5-7 minutes.
2. Add chopped bell pepper, carrot, and zucchini to the pot. Cook for another 5 minutes, stirring occasionally.
3. Stir in diced tomatoes, cumin, coriander, paprika, and cinnamon. Pour in water and bring the mixture to a boil.
4. Stir in quinoa, reduce heat to low, cover, and simmer for 30 minutes, or until the quinoa is cooked and most of the liquid is absorbed.
5. Season with salt and pepper. Garnish with chopped cilantro before serving.

Nutritional Information (per serving): Calories: 350

- Fat: 8g
- Saturated Fat: 1.5g
- Sodium: 200mg
- Carbohydrates: 40g
- Fiber: 5g
- Sugar: 6g
- Protein: 30g

Tips and Variations:

1. Add a handful of dried apricots or raisins for sweetness and texture.
2. Swap quinoa for couscous if not adhering strictly to a gluten-free diet.
3. Enhance the tagine with a splash of lemon juice for added zest.

Thai Green Curry with Chicken and Bamboo Shoots

Prep Time: 10 minutes

Cook Time: 20 minutes

Total Time: 30 minutes

Serving Size: 4 servings

Ingredients:

- 1 tablespoon coconut oil
- 1 lb. chicken breast, thinly sliced
- 2 tablespoons low FODMAP green curry paste (check ingredients to ensure no onion/garlic)
- 1 can (14 ounces) coconut milk
- 1 cup bamboo shoots, drained
- 1 bell pepper, sliced
- 1/2 cup green beans, trimmed
- 1 tablespoon fish sauce
- 1 teaspoon sugar
- Fresh basil leaves, for garnish

Instructions:

1. Heat coconut oil in a large skillet over medium heat. Add sliced chicken and sauté until cooked through, about 5-7 minutes.
2. Stir in green curry paste and cook for another minute until fragrant.

3. Pour in coconut milk and bring to a simmer. Add bamboo shoots, sliced bell pepper, and green beans.

4. Season with fish sauce and sugar. Let the curry simmer gently for 10-12 minutes or until the vegetables are tender and the flavors meld.

5. Serve hot, garnished with fresh basil leaves.

Nutritional Information (per serving): Calories: 300

- Fat: 18g

- Saturated Fat: 13g

- Sodium: 600mg

- Carbohydrates: 10g

- Fiber: 2g

- Sugar: 5g

- Protein: 25g

Tips and Variations:

1. Add slices of red chili or a squeeze of lime juice for an extra kick.

2. For a vegetarian version, substitute chicken with tofu and ensure the curry paste and fish sauce are suitable for vegetarians.

3. Serve over steamed jasmine rice or cauliflower rice for a complete meal.

Prep Time: 15 minutes (plus marinating time)

Cook Time: 10 minutes

Total Time: 25 minutes plus marinating

Serving Size: 4 servings

Ingredients:

- For the Lamb Kebabs:
- 1 lb lamb, cubed
- 2 tablespoons olive oil
- 1 teaspoon cumin
- 1 teaspoon smoked paprika
- 1/2 teaspoon dried mint
- Salt and pepper, to taste

For the Greek Salad:

- 3 cups mixed greens (romaine, arugula)
- 1 cucumber, diced
- 10 cherry tomatoes, halved
- 1/4 cup sliced black olives (ensure low FODMAP)
- 1/4 cup crumbled lactose-free feta cheese
- 2 tablespoons olive oil
- 1 tablespoon red wine vinegar
- Salt and pepper, to taste

Instructions:

1. In a bowl, mix olive oil, cumin, smoked paprika, dried mint, salt, and pepper. Add lamb cubes and stir to coat evenly. Marinate for at least 1 hour in the refrigerator.
2. Preheat grill to medium-high heat. Thread lamb onto skewers.
3. Grill kebabs for 8-10 minutes, turning occasionally, until cooked to desired doneness.
4. For the salad, combine mixed greens, cucumber, cherry tomatoes, black olives, and feta cheese in a large bowl.
5. In a small bowl, whisk together olive oil, red wine vinegar, salt, and pepper. Drizzle over the salad and toss to coat.
6. Serve kebabs alongside the fresh Greek salad.

Nutritional Information (per serving): Calories: 450

- Fat: 30g
- Saturated Fat: 10g
- Carbohydrates: 12g
- Fiber: 3g
- Sugar: 4g
- Protein: 35g

Tips and Variations:

1. Substitute lamb with chicken or beef if preferred.
2. Add a splash of lemon juice to the salad dressing for extra zest.
3. For a heartier salad, include quinoa or rice.

TASTY SNACK IDEAS

Pineapple Cottage Cheese (Lactose-Free)

Prep Time: 5 minutes

Total Time: 5 minutes

Serving Size: 1 serving

Ingredients:

- 1/2 cup lactose-free cottage cheese
- 1/2 cup diced pineapple (fresh or canned in its own juice)

Instructions:

1. Place the lactose-free cottage cheese in a serving bowl.
2. Top with diced pineapple.
3. Serve immediately or chill in the refrigerator before serving for extra freshness.

Nutritional Information (per serving): Calories: 180

- Fat: 2g
- Saturated Fat: 1g
- Sodium: 400mg
- Carbohydrates: 20g
- Fiber: 1g
- Sugar: 16g
- Protein: 16g

Tips and Variations:

1. Add a sprinkle of cinnamon or nutmeg for enhanced flavor.

2. Mix in other low FODMAP fruits like strawberries or blueberries for variety.

3. Drizzle with a little honey or maple syrup if a sweeter taste is desired.

Mixed Berry Fruit Salad

Prep Time: 10 minutes

Total Time: 10 minutes

Serving Size: 2 servings

Ingredients:

- 1/2 cup strawberries, sliced

- 1/2 cup blueberries

- 1/2 cup raspberries

- 1/2 cup blackberries

- Juice of 1/2 lemon

- Optional: 1 tablespoon chopped fresh mint for garnish

Instructions:

1. Combine strawberries, blueberries, raspberries, and blackberries in a large bowl.

2. Squeeze the juice of half a lemon over the berries and gently toss to combine.

3. Refrigerate until ready to serve.

4. Garnish with fresh mint before serving, if desired.

Nutritional Information (per serving): Calories: 90

- Fat: 0.5g

- Saturated Fat: 0g

- Sodium: 0mg

- Carbohydrates: 21g

- Fiber: 8g

- Sugar: 12g

- Protein: 2g

Tips and Variations:

1. Serve over lactose-free yogurt or ice cream for a decadent dessert.

2. Drizzle with a balsamic glaze for a gourmet touch.

3. Add a dollop of whipped coconut cream for a creamy texture.

Prep Time: 10 minutes

Total Time: 10 minutes

Serving Size: 2 servings

Ingredients:

- 1 carrot, peeled and cut into sticks
- 1 cucumber, cut into sticks
- 1 red bell pepper, cut into sticks
- 1/2 cup low FODMAP hummus (homemade or store-bought, ensuring no garlic or onion)

Instructions:

1. Arrange carrot, cucumber, and red bell pepper sticks on a plate.
2. Serve with a bowl of low FODMAP hummus for dipping.

Nutritional Information (per serving): Calories: 150

- Fat: 8g
- Saturated Fat: 1g
- Sodium: 300mg
- Carbohydrates: 18g
- Fiber: 5g
- Sugar: 6g
- Protein: 6g

Tips and Variations:

1. Add other veggies like radishes or green beans for more variety.

2. Sprinkle hummus with paprika or drizzle with olive oil for extra flavor.

3. For a zesty hummus, add lemon juice or a pinch of cayenne pepper.

Gluten-Free Crackers with Almond Butter and Banana

Prep Time: 5 minutes

Total Time: 5 minutes

Serving Size: 1 serving

Ingredients:

-   4 gluten-free crackers

-   2 tablespoons almond butter

-   1 small banana, sliced

Instructions:

1. Spread almond butter evenly on each gluten-free cracker.

2. Top each cracker with banana slices.

3. Serve immediately and enjoy.

Nutritional Information (per serving): Calories: 280

- Fat: 14g
- Saturated Fat: 2g
- Sodium: 200mg
- Carbohydrates: 36g
- Fiber: 5g
- Sugar: 14g
- Protein: 6g

Tips and Variations:

1. Substitute almond butter with peanut butter or sunflower seed butter.
2. Sprinkle with cinnamon or cocoa powder for added flavor.
3. Add a drizzle of honey or maple syrup for extra sweetness.

Prep Time: 5 minutes

Total Time: 5 minutes

Serving Size: 1 serving

Ingredients:

- 1 cup unsweetened almond milk
- 1 scoop low FODMAP protein powder (vanilla or unflavored)
- 1 small banana
- 1 tablespoon chia seeds

Instructions:

1. Combine almond milk, protein powder, banana, and chia seeds in a blender.
2. Blend on high until smooth.
3. Serve immediately, or chill in the refrigerator for a cold, refreshing drink.

Nutritional Information (per serving): Calories: 300

- Fat: 9g
- Saturated Fat: 1g
- Sodium: 180mg
- Carbohydrates: 34g
- Fiber: 7g

- Sugar: 14g
- Protein: 20g

Tips and Variations:

1. Add a handful of spinach or kale for extra nutrients without affecting the taste significantly.
2. Mix in a tablespoon of cocoa powder for a chocolatey version.
3. Use frozen banana to make the smoothie creamier and colder.

Lactose-Free Yogurt with Banana Slices

Prep Time: 5 minutes

Total Time: 5 minutes

Serving Size: 1 serving

Ingredients:

- 1 cup lactose-free yogurt
- 1 medium banana, sliced

Instructions:

1. Spoon the lactose-free yogurt into a serving bowl.
2. Top with freshly sliced banana.
3. Serve immediately for a refreshing and healthy snack.

Nutritional Information (per serving): Calories: 240

- Fat: 4g
- Saturated Fat: 2.5g
- Cholesterol: 15mg
- Sodium: 120mg
- Carbohydrates: 42g
- Fiber: 3g
- Sugar: 29g (includes natural sugars from the banana)
- Protein: 11g

Tips and Variations:

1. Sprinkle with a pinch of cinnamon or nutmeg for extra flavor.
2. Mix in a tablespoon of flaxseeds or chia seeds for added fiber and nutrients.
3. For an extra crunch, add a handful of gluten-free granola.

Prep Time: 2 minutes

Cook Time: 3 minutes

Total Time: 5 minutes

Serving Size: 2 servings

Ingredients:

- 1/4 cup popcorn kernels
- 1 tablespoon olive oil
- Salt, to taste

Instructions:

1. In a large pot, heat the olive oil over medium heat.
2. Add the popcorn kernels and cover with a lid.
3. Once the kernels start popping, shake the pot occasionally to prevent the popcorn from burning.
4. When the popping sound slows down, remove the pot from heat and keep covered until the popping stops.
5. Season with a dash of salt and serve hot.

Nutritional Information (per serving): Calories: 150

- Fat: 8g
- Saturated Fat: 1g
- Sodium: 290mg (varies with salt amount)
- Carbohydrates: 18g

- Fiber: 3g

- Sugar: 0g

- Protein: 2g

Tips and Variations:

1. For a sweet twist, toss the popcorn with a teaspoon of cinnamon and a sprinkle of sugar.

2. Add nutritional yeast after popping for a cheesy flavor without the dairy.

3. Experiment with different oils like coconut or avocado for varying flavors.

Cucumber and Carrot Sticks with Peanut Butter

Prep Time: 10 minutes

Total Time: 10 minutes

Serving Size: 2 servings

Ingredients:

- 1 large cucumber, cut into sticks

- 2 large carrots, peeled and cut into sticks

- 1/4 cup natural peanut butter

Instructions:

1. Wash and prepare the cucumber and carrots by cutting them into stick shapes suitable for dipping.

2. Serve the fresh cucumber and carrot sticks alongside a bowl of natural peanut butter for dipping.

3. Enjoy this crunchy and satisfying snack.

Nutritional Information (per serving): Calories: 180

- Fat: 12g

- Saturated Fat: 2.5g

- Sodium: 150mg

- Carbohydrates: 15g

- Fiber: 4g

- Sugar: 7g

- Protein: 6g

Tips and Variations:

1. Substitute peanut butter with almond butter or tahini for those with peanut allergies.

2. Sprinkle the peanut butter with a dash of cinnamon or cocoa powder for added flavor.

3. Add a drizzle of honey over the peanut butter for a touch of sweetness.

Prep Time: 5 minutes (plus chilling)

Cook Time: 5 minutes

Total Time: 2 hours 10 minutes

Serving Size: 4 servings

Ingredients:

- 1 package (0.3 ounces) sugar-free strawberry gelatin
- 1 cup boiling water
- 1 cup cold water

Instructions:

1. In a medium bowl, dissolve the strawberry gelatin in 1 cup of boiling water, stirring until completely dissolved.
2. Stir in 1 cup of cold water.
3. Pour the gelatin mixture into a serving dish or individual cups.
4. Refrigerate for at least 2 hours, or until the gelatin is firm and set.
5. Serve chilled.

Nutritional Information (per serving): Calories: 10

- Fat: 0g
- Saturated Fat: 0g
- Sodium: 35mg
- Carbohydrates: 0g
- Fiber: 0g

- Sugar: 0g
- Protein: 1g

Tips and Variations:

1. Add fresh strawberries or other low FODMAP fruits like blueberries for extra flavor and a nice visual appeal.
2. To make a layered gelatin dessert, partially set one layer before adding another layer of a different flavored gelatin.

Almond Butter Energy Balls

Prep Time: 15 minutes

Chill Time: 1 hour

Total Time: 1 hour 15 minutes

Serving Size: 12 balls

Ingredients:

- 1 cup rolled oats (ensure gluten-free if necessary)
- 1/2 cup almond butter
- 1/4 cup maple syrup
- 1/4 cup mini chocolate chips (ensure lactose-free if sensitive)
- 1/4 cup dried cranberries, chopped
- 1 tablespoon chia seeds

Instructions:

1. In a large mixing bowl, combine the rolled oats, almond butter, maple syrup, mini chocolate chips, chopped dried cranberries, and chia seeds.
2. Stir the mixture until all ingredients are well combined.
3. Using your hands, form the mixture into small balls, about 1 inch in diameter.
4. Place the energy balls on a baking sheet lined with parchment paper.
5. Refrigerate for at least 1 hour, or until the balls are firm.
6. Serve chilled or at room temperature.

Nutritional Information (per ball): Calories: 150

- Fat: 9g
- Saturated Fat: 1.5g
- Sodium: 10mg
- Carbohydrates: 16g
- Fiber: 2g
- Sugar: 9g
- Protein: 4g

Tips and Variations:

1. Substitute almond butter with peanut butter or sunflower seed butter for a different flavor.
2. Add a scoop of protein powder for an extra protein boost.
3. Roll the balls in coconut flakes or cocoa powder for an additional texture and flavor layer.

Prep Time: 10 minutes

Cook Time: 15 minutes

Total Time: 25 minutes

Serving Size: 4 servings

Ingredients:

- 6 corn tortillas
- 1 tablespoon olive oil
- Salt, to taste

For the Low FODMAP Salsa:

- 2 medium tomatoes, finely chopped
- 1/4 cup chopped green onion tops (green parts only)
- 1/4 cup chopped fresh cilantro
- 1 tablespoon lime juice
- Salt and pepper, to taste

Instructions:

1. Preheat your oven to 375°F (190°C).
2. Brush both sides of the corn tortillas with olive oil and sprinkle lightly with salt.
3. Cut the tortillas into wedges and spread them in a single layer on a baking sheet.
4. Bake in the preheated oven for 10-15 minutes, or until crisp and golden brown. Rotate the sheet halfway through for even baking.

5. Meanwhile, combine tomatoes, green onion tops, cilantro, and lime juice in a bowl. Season with salt and pepper to taste. Mix well to combine.

6. Serve the baked tortilla chips warm with the freshly made low FODMAP salsa.

Nutritional Information (per serving): Calories: 150

- Fat: 5g

- Saturated Fat: 0.5g

- Sodium: 120mg

- Carbohydrates: 24g

- Fiber: 4g

- Sugar: 2g

- Protein: 3g

Tips and Variations:

1. Add a pinch of cumin or smoked paprika to the tortilla chips before baking for extra flavor.

2. For a spicier salsa, add a small amount of chopped jalapeño (ensure tolerance).

Homemade Banana Bread (Gluten-Free)

Prep Time: 15 minutes

Cook Time: 1 hour

Total Time: 1 hour 15 minutes

Serving Size: 10 slices

Ingredients:

- 3 ripe bananas, mashed
- 1/3 cup melted coconut oil
- 1/2 cup maple syrup
- 2 eggs
- 1 teaspoon vanilla extract
- 1/2 teaspoon salt
- 1 teaspoon baking soda
- 1/2 teaspoon ground cinnamon
- 1 3/4 cups gluten-free all-purpose flour

Instructions:

1. Preheat the oven to 350°F (175°C). Grease a 9x5 inch loaf pan.
2. In a large bowl, mix mashed bananas with melted coconut oil. Stir in maple syrup, eggs, and vanilla extract.
3. Add salt, baking soda, and cinnamon. Mix in the gluten-free flour until just combined.
4. Pour the batter into the prepared loaf pan.
5. Bake for 60 minutes, or until a toothpick inserted into the center comes out clean.

6. Let cool in the pan for 10 minutes, then turn out onto a wire rack to cool completely before slicing.

Nutritional Information (per slice): Calories: 230

- Fat: 9g
- Saturated Fat: 6g
- Sodium: 240mg
- Carbohydrates: 37g
- Fiber: 3g
- Sugar: 17g
- Protein: 3g

Tips and Variations:

1. Add chocolate chips or nuts for additional texture and flavor.
2. Swap maple syrup with honey or another sweetener if preferred.
3. Serve toasted with a smear of lactose-free butter or peanut butter.

MANAGING IBS LONG-TERM

Beyond the Low FODMAP Diet: Other Lifestyle Factors

While the Low FODMAP Diet is a crucial tool in managing Irritable Bowel Syndrome (IBS), it's important to recognize that long-term management often requires a more holistic approach. Lifestyle factors such as stress management, regular exercise, and adequate sleep play significant roles in the overall health and well-being of individuals with IBS. Integrating these elements can enhance the effectiveness of dietary changes and lead to better symptom control and quality of life.

Stress Management Techniques

1. **Mindfulness and Meditation:** Regular practice of mindfulness and meditation can significantly reduce stress levels, which in turn can alleviate IBS symptoms. Techniques like guided imagery, mindfulness-based stress reduction (MBSR), and breathing exercises help calm the mind and reduce the body's stress response.

2. **Cognitive Behavioral Therapy (CBT):** CBT is an effective tool for managing chronic illness, including IBS. It helps modify negative thoughts and behaviors related to stress and anxiety, providing strategies to cope with the emotional aspects of living with IBS.

3. **Yoga and Relaxation:** Yoga combines physical postures, breathing exercises, and meditation to enhance relaxation and stress management. Specific yoga poses can also help with digestion and alleviate abdominal discomfort.

Importance of Regular Exercise

1. Enhancing Digestive Health: Regular physical activity helps increase the efficiency of the digestive system. It can speed up the transit time of food in the digestive tract, which is beneficial for those with IBS, particularly for those prone to constipation.

2. Reducing Stress: Exercise is a natural stress reliever. Activities like walking, cycling, swimming, or team sports not only improve physical health but also help reduce anxiety and depression, which can exacerbate IBS symptoms.

3. Improving Overall Well-being: Regular exercise boosts energy levels, helps in maintaining a healthy weight, and improves overall body image, which can positively affect how individuals manage their IBS.

Getting Adequate Sleep

1. Impact on Gut Health: There is a two-way relationship between sleep and gut health. Poor sleep can exacerbate gastrointestinal symptoms, while IBS symptoms can also lead to disrupted sleep. Maintaining a regular sleep schedule helps regulate the body's internal clock, which can improve digestive health.

2. Sleep Hygiene Practices: Good sleep hygiene practices are essential for quality sleep. These include maintaining a consistent sleep schedule, creating a restful environment (dark, quiet, and cool), avoiding caffeine and heavy meals close to bedtime, and disconnecting from electronic devices at least an hour before sleep.

3. Managing Pain and Discomfort: For those whose IBS symptoms flare up at night, it might be helpful to adopt positions that ease discomfort. For example, sleeping on one's left side can reduce acid reflux, and using a body pillow can provide extra support and comfort.

Combining Approaches for Optimal Management

Successfully managing IBS long-term often requires combining dietary management with these lifestyle modifications. Each person's response to these changes can vary, so it's important to adopt a personalized approach, perhaps starting with one or two changes and gradually incorporating more as needed.

Furthermore, ongoing support from healthcare professionals, such as gastroenterologists, dietitians, and mental health therapists, can provide guidance and encouragement throughout this process. By addressing not only the physical but also the emotional and psychological aspects of IBS, individuals can achieve a better quality of life and more effective control over their symptoms.

Long-Term Dietary Maintenance

To effectively manage IBS over the long term, maintaining a healthy gut microbiome and ensuring adequate intake of fiber and probiotics are crucial. These components not only support digestive health but also enhance overall wellbeing. Here are key strategies to help you maintain these important aspects of your diet.

Strategies for Maintaining a Healthy Gut Microbiome

1. Diverse Diet: Once you've identified your FODMAP thresholds, aim to reintroduce a wide variety of foods into your diet. A diverse diet can help nourish a diverse microbiome, which is beneficial for overall gut health. Include plenty of different fruits, vegetables, grains, and proteins that are tolerable to your system.

2. Fermented Foods: Include foods that naturally contain beneficial bacteria, such as yogurt, kefir, sauerkraut, kimchi, and kombucha. These can help increase the diversity and number of beneficial microbes in your gut. Ensure that these fermented foods are low in FODMAPs and fit within your tolerance levels.

3. Prebiotic Foods: Prebiotics are types of dietary fiber that feed the good bacteria in your gut. Foods like bananas, onions, garlic, leeks, asparagus, and whole grains contain prebiotics. However, since some prebiotic foods are high in FODMAPs, reintroduce them cautiously and monitor your symptoms.

Incorporating Fiber in Your Diet

1. Gradual Increase: If you have been on a restricted diet, it's important to gradually increase fiber intake to prevent any abrupt digestive discomfort. Start with soluble fiber sources, which are easier on the gut, such as oats, carrots, berries, and peeled fruits.

2. Balanced Fiber Sources: Aim to include both soluble and insoluble fiber in your diet. Soluble fiber, found in foods like oats, nuts, seeds, and legumes, helps to soften stools, which can ease constipation. Insoluble fiber, found in whole grains and vegetables, adds bulk to the stool and can help with bowel regularity.

3. Hydration: As you increase your fiber intake, also increase your fluid intake. Water helps fiber do its job by adding bulk to the stool and making it easier to pass, thus reducing the risk of constipation.

Probiotics for Gut Health

1. Probiotic Supplements: Consider incorporating a probiotic supplement, especially if your diet does not allow for much variety in fermented foods. Supplements can help maintain or restore a healthy balance of gut bacteria. It's important to choose a probiotic that is evidence-based and suited for managing IBS symptoms, such as those containing Bifidobacteria and Lactobacilli strains.

2. Regular Consumption: For probiotics to be effective, they need to be taken regularly. These beneficial bacteria do not permanently colonize the gut but can influence the overall health of the microbiome while they are present.

3. Consultation with a Healthcare Provider: Before starting any probiotic supplement, especially if you have a complex or severe gastrointestinal condition, consult with a healthcare provider. They can provide guidance on the best types and strains of probiotics for your specific condition.

Monitoring and Adjusting Your Diet

Maintaining a healthy gut involves regular monitoring of your diet and symptoms, and possibly adjusting your intake of fibers, probiotics, and various food groups based on how your symptoms evolve. As your gut health improves or as your body changes, your dietary needs might shift as well.

By adopting these strategies, you can help ensure that your diet supports a healthy gut microbiome, aids in managing your IBS symptoms, and contributes to your overall health and wellbeing. Remember, each individual's needs can vary, so it's beneficial to tailor these recommendations to fit your specific health profile and dietary tolerances.

Seeking Support and Resources

Managing Irritable Bowel Syndrome (IBS) is not just about adhering to dietary guidelines; it's also about navigating the emotional and practical challenges that come with a chronic condition. Support and resources are crucial for maintaining motivation, obtaining useful information, and enhancing your coping strategies. Here's how you can tap into various types of support and utilize resources effectively.

Joining Support Groups

1. Benefits of Support Groups: Support groups provide a platform to share experiences, tips, and encouragement with others who understand what you're going through. They can offer emotional support, reduce feelings of isolation, and provide a sense of community.

2. Finding the Right Group: Look for local or online IBS support groups. Many organizations and hospitals run regular support group meetings. Online forums and social media groups offer flexibility and accessibility, allowing you to connect with peers globally.

3. Active Participation: Actively participating in these groups can enhance your understanding of IBS management strategies that work for others and might work for you. Sharing your own experiences can also be cathartic and helpful to others.

Utilizing Online Resources and Apps

1. Educational Websites: Websites such as those run by gastrointestinal health organizations, like the International Foundation for Gastrointestinal Disorders (IFFGD) or the Monash University FODMAP website, provide reliable information, research updates, and practical tips for managing IBS.

2. Mobile Apps: Apps like the Monash University FODMAP app can help you track your diet, identify low and high FODMAP foods, and monitor your symptoms. Other apps designed for stress reduction and mindfulness, such as Headspace or Calm, can also be beneficial in managing the stress component of IBS.

3. Blogs and Podcasts: Many health professionals and individuals with IBS run blogs and podcasts, sharing their insights and coping mechanisms. These can offer new perspectives and practical advice that can be integrated into your daily routine.

Communicating with Your Healthcare Provider

1. Regular Check-Ins: Schedule regular appointments with your healthcare provider to discuss your progress, challenges, and any adjustments needed in your treatment plan. These check-ins are crucial for tracking the effectiveness of your management strategies.

2. Preparing for Appointments: To make the most of your appointments, prepare a list of questions or concerns beforehand. Keep a diary of your symptoms, diet, and any non-dietary factors that affect your IBS, such as stress or sleep patterns.

3. Collaborative Approach: Consider your relationship with your healthcare provider as a partnership. Be open about what's working and what isn't, and discuss various approaches to manage your condition, including changes in diet, lifestyle adjustments, and mental health support.

4. Specialist Referrals: If your symptoms are complex or difficult to manage, ask for referrals to specialists such as gastroenterologists, dietitians, or mental health professionals who have experience dealing with IBS.

Leveraging these support systems and resources can significantly enhance your ability to manage IBS effectively. Whether it's through connecting with others in a similar situation, utilizing digital tools to keep track of your diet and symptoms, or maintaining open communication with your healthcare team, each step you take is crucial in building a comprehensive support system that caters to all aspects of living with IBS.

CONCLUSION

As you reach the end of this journey through the complexities of managing Irritable Bowel Syndrome (IBS) with the Low FODMAP Diet, it's essential to reflect on the key concepts we've explored together and to look forward with hope and determination.

Throughout this book, we've looked into the intricacies of IBS, understanding its symptoms, its impact on daily life, and the challenges it presents. We've embraced the Low FODMAP Diet as a powerful tool for managing symptoms, learning about FODMAPs, and navigating the phases of elimination, reintroduction, and personalization.

Beyond dietary considerations, we've explored the importance of lifestyle factors such as stress management, regular exercise, and adequate sleep in maintaining gut health and overall well-being. We've discussed strategies for incorporating fiber and probiotics, nurturing a healthy gut microbiome, and seeking support and resources to guide you on your journey.

As you move forward, remember that managing IBS is a journey, not a destination. There will be ups and downs, challenges and victories, but with each step, you are gaining valuable insight into your body and how to support it. Embrace the journey with patience and resilience, knowing that you are not alone.

Reach out to support groups, utilize online resources, and maintain open communication with your healthcare provider. Empower yourself with knowledge, listen to your body, and trust your instincts. You have the strength within you to navigate this path and to live a fulfilling life despite the challenges of IBS.

Above all, be kind to yourself. Celebrate your successes, no matter how small, and be gentle with yourself during setbacks. Remember that you are more than your condition, and you deserve compassion, understanding, and support.

As you embark on the next chapter of your journey, may you find relief, resilience, and renewed vitality. You are capable, you are courageous, and you are not alone. Here's to your health, happiness, and a future filled with possibilities. Keep moving forward, one step at a time. You've got this.